Table of Contents

I0408167

Dedication

I dedicate this book to my best friend Donnell who has been my number one fan since the 7th grade and has been encouraging me to write it for the past 10 years. Well here it is D!

Introduction

I first became aware of my hair when I was five or six years old in kindergarten during a school picture and as we were preparing for the photo two older girls behind me were openly discussing my hair. My mom had put my hair into ponytails that morning but I guess the naps on the back of my neck made for a very interesting topic amongst the girls. I didn't say anything nor did I turn around but I remember feeling very bad and it was the beginning of me feeling self-conscious about how my hair looked to other people.

Growing up I always noticed how the other girls hair looked in comparison to mine. The girls at school had hair that was impeccably neat and that could have been due to the fact that they had sisters at home to help them every morning or maybe they were able to do it themselves I don't know but I was painfully aware of the fact that I did not have hair that was as neat or long as theirs. Don't get me wrong my mother did what she knew how to do but it wasn't consistent and because I looked at myself every day, I couldn't help but notice.

Around 11 or 12 years old I basically stopped allowing my mother to do my hair. Although she would sometimes take me to the salon with her to get my hair done, I would have to get a haircut and when I left the salon, there were no hair care instructions given to me at my age so I didn't know how to take care of my hair. I had absolutely no knowledge about the damage that was being done with the relaxers that were put on my hair or how it was drying out from a lack of product and proper maintenance. It's just my opinion but girls that are 13 and under should not necessarily have hairstyles that they are unable to maintain. It's such an impressionable age and you're dealing with so many insecurities about how you look. It's also when you start developing and dealing with acne plus your limbs are not all in proportion with the rest of your body. There's just so much going on that constantly make you feel weird and the last thing a young girl needs is to feel unattractive because her hair isn't looking right. Kids are very cruel and will make sure you feel worse if you are looking bad to them.

At 15 years old , I was going to a school dance and one of my girlfriend's brother agreed to be my date. My grandmother helped me with my dress and I was on my own with my hair and didn't have any makeup so I don't believe I wore any but I did the best I knew how to do to make myself look presentable. Anyway we get there and when it's time to take photos, I see from across the room that everyone is talking to him and based on what I could see he did not want to take a picture with me. I didn't understand this but the only thing I could sum up was he wasn't happy with how I looked and didn't want to be seen with me because in LA at that time, it was all about the light-skinned girls with the "water and lotion hair" and I definitely wasn't one of those. I don't even remember if we wound up taking the photo but it was a very embarrassing experience for me and as you can see by this recount, it is one that I have not forgotten.

Up to this point I had already been through ponytails, cornrows, Jheri curls, and relaxers so after this ordeal my mother had someone put individual braids into my hair. I remember the lady working very long hours on me well past midnight into the next morning and when my grandmother picked me up, I don't even think my mother had all of this woman's money to pay for the service which bothered me so much to the point that I continued to question my mom about whether or not she gave the lady the final payment on my hair. Mainly because I knew if my hair wasn't paid for then I wouldn't be unable to go back to her and get it done again. After my hair grew out, I sat down one day and took the braids out one at a time and replaced them until my entire head was completely re-braided. This, at least allowed me to keep a neat appearance until I could figure something else out.

During the second semester in the 10th grade my mother moved us out of LA and into East Valley where I experienced extreme culture shock in La Puente California but I can honestly say I had a good time there. Anyway this is when I started making a little money on my own braiding the hair of other girls at the school so I could have a little pocket change to buy hair of my own to keep my hair braided. It's so funny because the quality of human hair that I bought wasn't always the best and I found myself constantly having to spray it with water and conditioner so it wouldn't get all big and puffy. I look back on it now as one big nuisance because no one should have to pay that much attention to their hair while in school or at work or while doing anything for that matter, but that's what it was so I dealt with it.

By the age of 18, I had discovered hair weaving that I gladly displayed in my senior prom although it was just a couple of pieces in the front to give me some long bangs, but I soon learned how to put my own hair weave in and from then on I was hooked. It was a way for me to have different looks without having to be bothered with my own hair and when I was ready to grow out of my relaxer, that is the way I chose to do it because then I didn't have to deal with two different textures while going through that transitional phase. I would shampoo, condition, trim my ends and put the hair weave back in. This was my routine for at least two years until the early 90s when I would get my hair pressed because I felt it was long enough to wear out.

After high school I enrolled in cosmetology school so I could pursue a career that would allow me the flexibility to move around and be my own boss without having someone else tell me what to do. I went to school full-time during the day and worked as a waitress at night to pay for my tuition and lived off of my tips as far as what I ate while I was out of the house. I believe I moved five times in 10 months because I didn't have the tools necessary to teach me how to be on my own so I was at the mercy of wherever my mother was living and or whoever would take me in. I temporarily lived with my father while I was in cosmetology school and commuted to school at 6 AM, got out of school at 4:00 PM and went straight to work by 5 PM not getting off until 12 or 1 AM in the morning. My commute in the morning was usually an hour because I was living in LA and working and going to school in East Valley. It was indeed a hard 10 months because my living arrangements were unstable and I was trying to pursue a career no one really supported. There wasn't much interest taken in my education so this was the only way I knew how to take charge of what I wanted to do in my life. I don't feel anyone was necessarily against what I wanted to do just not interested.

During that time I would go between braids and getting it pressed but pretty much staying in that whole natural and chemical free phase of my hair care. By this time, I had grown tired of purchasing hair and walking around with someone else's DNA on my head and losing extensions on the dance floor because my braids weren't tight enough and trying to hide my tracks so guys wouldn't see that my hair was fake. That in itself was a full-time job so I retired the hair weaves and the braids for good along with the pressing comb and the burnt hair smell to go into something a little less expensive so to speak.

I started my first set of locks around 1997 and actually got the idea for how I started them from the girl I worked with in a braid shop in Decatur Georgia. She was from Senegal and taught me how to do Senegalese twists which is what we call two strand twist today. At a natural hair care show in Atlanta, I met the sister lock owner and her twin sisters as they were displaying the interlock method she used to create a tiny lock that wouldn't break like it would from traditional palm rolling. I considered the interlock method for myself but I didn't want to rely on someone else to do my hair and I didn't want to spend that much time doing my hair. I preferred the look of a palm rolled lock because it's a much smoother look and the hair does what it needs to do on its own and not from me creating it through a braid using a tool the way the interlock method does because it's just a backwards braid without hair added in. Palm rolling allows the hair to loc naturally where interlocking produces a manufactured loc that is created by braiding the hair with a tool for those who don't know the difference. The choice between the two methods would be a matter of preference on the part of the individual. With that being said, I two strand twisted my own hair and didn't comb it out for two weeks and found that the hair matted very quickly within a three week period so I merely shampooed it while it was twisted and then re-twisted it until it was time for it to be palm rolled and it allowed me to bypass a messy or fuzzy look while I was going through the locking process.

I've been through every style imaginable and some of those experiences with my hair were embarrassing, depressing and even painful, but I'm glad I had those experiences because it taught me a lot. With the knowledge that I've gained over the years I am able to share that information with other people that are struggling with their hair issues especially since we are in a new age of natural hair. No longer is it embarrassing or considered country or uncultured to wear your hair natural; it is embraced and considered beautiful. I hope that whoever reads this information will walk away with something valuable because it is my goal not only to inform but to encourage and motivate others to simply be who they are.

Chapter 1

Salon Etiquette for Stylists

In this section I'd like to point out some things that get the most attention in terms of complaints from clients. Although you can't please everybody, I do feel some of the gripes are valid and at one time I was guilty of one or more of these violations. Since I've grown in my business, I've developed a certain level of professionalism that allow me to attract mainly a business clientele. Keep in mind there are all types of stylists that draw all types of clientele and every client isn't good for every stylist so as I write this I'm aware that some of these practices just don't apply to everyone in the industry.

Time Management

It's no secret that things have changed in the hair care industry. Although it's a billion-dollar business, it is now dominated by Asian owned businesses with the majority of the consumers being African-American women. Another way the business has suffered is through the lack of professionalism from some stylists and unfortunately as artists, stylists tend to concentrate more on the creativity of the craft and not on the business side. Time management and people management skills seem to be a practice that's nonexistent in the hair world. It is a common complaint of consumers that they have to wait all day to get their hair done and when they finally get to the chair they may or may not receive the service they paid for. Now in defense of the hair stylist, overbooking is common due to client no-shows and last-minute cancellations that usually result in a loss of income for the stylist so to lessen the impact of this, hair stylists just schedule people as they want to come in order not to lose money. I'm not saying this is a good practice but that's why it is done and this is where people management skills come into play. If clients know up front that your time is valuable to you they will respect your time, but as a professional it is imperative that the stylists lead by example. Too often stylists will schedule an appointment in the morning let's say at 8 AM and show up at 8:15 (I used to be guilty of this) or even 8:30 AM leaving the client waiting. Now what that does is it instills in the client's mind that they too can show up around 8:15 AM and not be prompt because that is the behavior that the stylist has originally displayed to the client. It sends a message to the client that their time isn't valuable therefore your time isn't valuable. The rules of time management hasn't changed and are still the same. Being early is on time, being on time is late, and being late is disrespectful. Usually people with poor time management are late everywhere they go. They are late for their hair appointments, they're late picking their kids up from school, they're late for work, they're always rushing trying to get to the next destination because they don't manage their time well. When it comes to the clients that I deal with, I have found that the ones that are late are the same few people that are always late with a different excuse. That's how I identify the clients with poor time management because the ones that are on time are always on time no matter what the weather is like or how much traffic there is on the highway. When these people are late, there's a good reason for it (like a car accident). Yeah, something that drastic! I am very particular about time because I used to be a person with poor time management and was always late at least five minutes sometimes more and rushing to do things at the last minute because I was a chronic procrastinator and because I recognize myself as a procrastinator, I have to be early in order to be on time for any given appointment whether it's for me or for one of my clients. While working in Arizona a client of mine was waiting on me and I strolled in a few minutes late and during the appointment her husband spoke to me about my time management. For some reason, what he said concerning that topic, really stuck with me and ever since then I've been very aware of my own ability to be on time for appointments. I realized I was giving them permission to disrespect my time because I wasn't respecting them or the time that they took to come and patronize my business. My being on time encourages my clients to do the same and allows me to have a life outside of the salon instead of working in the salon all night because my schedule is backed up.

Maintain A Clean Work Environment

One of the things I make an effort to be conscious of, is my work environment and how clean it is. I make it a point to clean up after every client so that the last person coming in won't feel like they're on the tail end of the workday. Technically they are but the work environment doesn't have to reflect that. It's extremely important for your clientele to feel comfortable in the place where they're coming to get their hair done in order for them to be motivated to come back because the money is in a client's longevity not in the day-to-day hustle of getting people into the salon.

It's also important to keep all equipment such as combs, brushes and clippers properly sanitized to avoid spreading any infections to clients not to mention it protects the stylists from a hefty fine from state board if they were to come in and inspect the salon. Believe it or not, customers do pay attention to how much dust you have in the corner of your station, how much buildup there may be on top of your station and whether or not you are organized and tidy. They see all that and for some people a dirty salon is more than enough to keep them from coming back to you. Now some people just don't care and a little bit of a mess is probably neater then how they're living at home so all they want you to do is make sure their hair looks right before they leave the salon.

Put Salon Policies In Place

There are times when stylists are uncomfortable about reminding a client of a policy that exists in the salon for fear that the client may not come back, but when you put policies in place for the clients to follow, it actually creates a more professional environment because they know what they can or cannot do up front. This eliminates the uncomfortable task of having to ask the client to step outside to use their phone or take their child outside if they are noisy, etc. In a group setting where there are multiple stylists, it becomes the job of the owner to ensure that all employees or independent contractors inform their clients of salon policy.

Some salons allow children and some salons do not allow children. Years ago, I had to have my daughter in the salon with me and I think now I am a little traumatized by that. Don't get me wrong because she's was a shop baby and she knew how to be seen and not heard but nonetheless, it's not a good look to have your child at work with you. Luckily I was in a suite and I could keep her contained and out of site, but today I prefer not to have children on my job where I'm handling hot tools, sharp objects, and dealing with chemicals and sprays. It's truly an unsafe environment for children and they don't even like being in a salon setting anyway. My motto is this "I won't bring my child to your job so don't bring yours to mine". People tend to forget that we are at work and despite how it looks, it requires some form of concentration. If you're in a salon that is kid friendly, then there is usually a space designated for them. Also keep in mind that the salon owner has to have business insurance and if someone gets hurt in the salon, this can result in a claim that raises the owner's insurance.

Image and Hygiene

Image - Have you ever gotten to the salon and questioned the stylist's ability to do your hair based on how she looked? Looking busted on the job is poor representation of the business pure and simple. I don't know about other people, but I don't want anyone who looks sloppy to work on me in the beauty industry because I make an effort to keep my appearance together. Although there are days where I don't feel I look my best, I'm clean and my hair is usually neat. It doesn't matter whether I'm getting my nails done, a massage or whatever the service may be. Pay attention to how the person performing the service keeps themselves and yes this can affect whether or not I patronize them are not. This is just my opinion, but my logic behind this is, if they don't care about how they look then that lack of caring will show up somewhere along the line during one of my services. I don't expect anyone to agree with me, I'm merely giving my reason for feeling the way I do.

Hygiene - There's a phrase that says the block is hot well there's nothing hotter than a stylist's breath who hasn't eaten all day! I for one try to make an effort to spare my clients from such an unpleasant experience by keeping mints at my disposal. I admit sometimes I may be unsuccessful but I do check myself to make sure the next person doesn't have to suffer. Also, be conscious of body odor. I've worked on clients that didn't smell so good and there's just no tactful way to tell someone they have a body odor. As beauty professionals, we not only have to keep our appearances up on the outside but it is important to be conscious of what we put into our bodies plus practice proper hygiene in order not to offend our clientele. There's nothing wrong with a little freshening up when your deodorant has left the building.

Be Professional

It seems like a simple term but unfortunately some people don't know what it means to be professional. This isn't really a put down, just an observation I've made over the years while working with other stylists. Here are some things that would be considered unprofessional in my industry or any other industry that deals with the business of handling money in exchange for services.

Fights and arguments - As artists, stylists can be a bit flamboyant, egotistical, temperamental, and eccentric so drama in the salon is not an uncommon thing, but physical or verbal altercations in front of clients would be considered unprofessional. Although there are times when someone catches you on the wrong day and a spontaneous chin check becomes necessary.

Eating while working - I can understand if you're busy and you want to munch on a cracker or something just to knock the edge off the hunger but to be behind a client eating a sandwich or any other food is just not necessary. I mean really take a break already!

Drinking alcohol - some stylists like to serve wine to their clients but if the stylist is in the back making mixed drinks and coming back to the chair to try and work, it can very well affect their performance not to mention slow them down because alcohol is a depressant and you will not work at full capacity while under the influence.

Spouses or significant others - being in a partnership with your mate is one thing but having a girlfriend, boyfriend, wife or husband hanging out in the salon while a stylist is trying to work doesn't look good in front of the clients. By hanging out I mean being in the salon on a regular basis with nothing else to do other than count their significant other's money. In my opinion, based on life experience and observation, I feel it's best to keep clients out of your personal life as much as possible.

Conversations - whether you're on the cell phone while working or talking to someone over your clients head with someone who's just visiting, it's best to limit this type of activity so your client won't feel like you're not paying attention to them. The beauty industry is about pampering and clients want to feel like they're getting their money's worth by having their stylists or beauty professional pay full attention to them and having outside conversations while working for long periods of time can be considered rude to the client.

Don't Cheat The Client

There are different ways to cheat a client and stylists who have done it know exactly where I'm going with this and let's face it, people are not always honest. Some things are done out of necessity when the ends aren't meeting and some things are done because he or she is just a foul individual.

Putting cheap products in a professional product's bottle - So you run out of the good stuff and you put something less expensive in its place because you're already under charging the client and you can't afford to purchase a quality brand. This makes clients nervous if it has happened to them so buy what you can buy and make an effort not to mislead them

Performing services with limited skills - Know your limits and don't work on people to get the money because the real money is in customer retention anyway. During this natural hair care evolution, natural stylists are popping up everywhere and too many of them don't know what the hell they are doing. Not all naturalists are without knowledge and skill, but enough of them exist for me to take notice since I've had to fix enough mistakes to piss me off at this point. Some of the responsibility falls on the client too; I mean do your research because being in the salon doesn't automatically mean the stylist knows what they're doing even if they are licensed. Don't allow a person with a relaxer to twist your locs…REALLY! I shouldn't even have to put this in writing, but how are they going to relate to what's going on with your hair when they're still knowingly putting a poison on their scalp in order to straighten their hair? Beware of a stylist whose hair is almost never done, unhealthy or falling out. If they can't take care of their own hair, what makes you think they can take care of yours?

The cost of service doesn't match quality of service - A client comes in and wants a service you don't do that often such as locs or loc styling. Your skills are good enough to twist even though you may take all day, but the style is less than your best and the client doesn't appear to be too happy, but you charge them a hefty fee anyway. Not cool……Times are difficult and challenging for most people, but be fare. If a style is going south on me because I over estimated my skills at that moment then I will back off of the style and let the client know what's going on and do something that will yield a positive result because if they're happy I'm happy.

Salon Etiquette for Clients

There's a lot of emphasis put on finding a good stylist, but are you a good client? In my experience, I've come across some clients whose business just wasn't worth the money. As stylists, we are nothing without our clients, but that doesn't give anyone the green light to treat us like servants they can kick around. Believe it or not, what we do takes concentration, knowledge and skill and if everyone had the same skills, our jobs wouldn't exist. There are some who have a license, but lack the creativity to be an artist in this field…....unfortunately, but it's up to clients to do their research before allowing someone to work on their hair. For the sake of humor, here are some things that might make someone a "PC" (Problem Client) or a "PITA" (Pain In The Ass) in my opinion of course and the opinion of stylists who won't say it out loud, but discuss the topic amongst themselves. I've toned it down for the sake of my daughter who was all in her feelings when she read some of it therefore please don't take this section too seriously; it's meant to be funny so lighten up!

Mistaking the Beautician for a Magician…"surely there's a magic wand amongst those combs"

By the way, don't call us beauticians……Everyone wants beautiful healthy hair, but that doesn't happen in just one visit to the salon. It is a process that involves a healthy diet, stress management, and a hair care regimen implemented on a regular basis. Clients sometimes look at photos of styles they want to walk out with, but it's really only a style they can work toward. Women are notorious for choosing styles they don't have enough hair for and now that so many women are going back to their natural state, unrealistic expectations are high. Don't get me wrong, there's nothing wrong with having high expectations but know your limits. Also, I would like to add, that being natural doesn't mean you don't go get your hair done. Some women are taking the natural hair evolution a little too far waking up fluffing up their hair and walking outside as if it looks good and it doesn't always look good. Just my professional opinion of course. As women we should always be conscious of our appearance when we go in public and I am very happy that so many women have embraced their natural hair and not treating it like it's some sort of disease they don't want to catch but really! The bush look does not go well on everyone. What you see in a magazine is just that, a fashion photo shoot and it doesn't mean the look you see is the one you should be wearing when you go to work.

Being late almost every appointment…"I know I am 30 minutes late but I have some place to be in an hour"

Things happen and being late is a possibility. In defense of the client, stylists are well known for running behind, but that's usually because the stylist has poor time management and or the client has poor time management. This is something I had to learn because there is no reason to be late every appointment. The rule of time is as follows: 1. Early is on time, 2. On time is late and 3. Late is disrespectful. A client who is late every appointment is showing blatant disrespect for your time. And sometimes we get caught up in our own lives and **subconsciously** we think our time is more important than someone else's. Especially in the hair profession where people don't even see what we do as a real job.

elling your stylist what to do, when to do it, and how to do it..... "This is how my mom do my hair"

I had a client whose sister called in for her brother who wanted his hair done. I didn't find out he'd already been to a stylist that day until I got started, which is a red flag and is a sign of a 'chair jumper" which are people who say they know what they want but usually don't so they go from stylist to stylist not getting what they want because they're either never satisfied or constantly interfere with the work of the stylist. Anyway, the young man gets to the salon and proceeds to tell me how his mother does his hair and I thought to myself "Is this boy trying tell me to do a home job on his hair?! The answer to that is yes he was; He wasn't used to going to the salon and was unfamiliar with different methods used to get a natural style. He showed me a photo of what he wanted (which didn't look professional at all and should have been my first clue he was going to be a problem), but his hair was too short to achieve that look and of course I told him so, but he insisted on his hair being done the way his mother did it. Well I tried to comply (shame on me because I know better) and the style didn't turn out the way he wanted, but guess who got blamed? ME! To all the professionals out there, stick to what you know and don't allow anyone to disrespect your art. Letting you know the look they wish to achieve is all the client has to do and HOW it gets done is your department. The Internet got people messed up in the head and now everyone thinks they can do hair. On the flip side, hats off to those who are not professionally trained and do a great job in the kitchen, on the porch or in their garage. There are some people who may not be licensed, but are very good at doing hair but that does not include everyone. I'm all for getting information and educating oneself on the products that are used on their hair but getting too involved in the process of the service is taking it a little too far. If you've chosen an individual as a professional to provide a service for you, micromanaging the appointment will interfere with the stylist's ability to create. Quite frankly I don't want someone who's on my head to be irritated because of something I'm doing or saying to them. People tend to underestimate the power of touch and how it can affect them physically and emotionally and we must remember that energy is transferred and not destroyed. The results of an irritated stylist just might show up in your hair style or lack of hair style.

Pretending salon policy doesn't exist...."These rules don't apply to me anyway"

One of the salon policies I'm very strict about is cell phones. It is so rude to speak on your cell phone inside of a business where other people can hear you especially if it's an establishment where people are trying to relax. I don't want to hear another person's conversation while I'm trying to work so I ask clients to step outside if they must use their cell phones or answer calls because it interferes with the conversation I'm trying to have with the client that's in the chair and if they're in the chair, sure they may need to answer the phone to check on their kids or maybe it's a work call, but casual conversations don't necessarily need to be everyone's business. We can follow all the rules in other businesses but for some reason when it comes to a black-owned business, we want those rules not to apply to us and it isn't fair to the person attempting to be professional. There's no need to bring an entourage with you to your appointment, and although I've experienced not having a sitter, the salon is not a day care. Don't bring a child that needs to sit in your lap or crowd the work place with a stroller. We work with chemicals, sharp objects, and hot tools so the last thing we need is for anyone to crowd us unnecessarily especially if they are not being serviced. If you must bring people with you, have them wait in a waiting area designated for them.

Wanting the most while paying the least..." That price is a little high can't you just hook me up?"

I'm all for giving complementary services every once in a while, but coming into the salon without all your money to pay for services received is just out of line. We work on our feet, we have to pay to go to work, buy all our supplies and someone coming in not having their funds readily available or expecting to pay nothing such is the case with family who thinks being related to you gives them a free pass to use you, once services are rendered is enough to invoke a little violence within the stylist especially if you have worked all day. Also, wanting so much more then what you can afford to pay for is just out-of-pocket and in layman's terms, that shit ain't right. Some of you may say some services are too high or not worth the money but maybe it's just that it's not within your current budget. Always remember that you truly get what you pay for so if you don't want to pay or can't pay, then minimize your expectations.

Be hygienically correct..." What's that smell? I've been smelling it all day!"

Because it's coming from you! First of all, it takes so much more for a woman to be clean than it does for a man because of all the extra things we have going on every month and if we don't have the extra things going on every month then getting old is enough. Occasionally, you may not feel as fresh as you want to, but becoming nose blind to how you are smelling around your lady parts and other areas with holes in it is inexcusable. Body odor is considered offensive (here in the states anyway) so my suggestion for women who may have this issue is to simply soak in the tub. If you are heavy coffee drinkers or eat a lot of fast food it's going to affect how you smell when you go to the bathroom and although reading this may be a sensitive topic for people, I wouldn't be writing it if this hadn't been an experience of mine. Again, I try to reference myself because hell sometimes I may not smell so great after working all day, but I am conscious of it and do make the effort to correct it. Next let's discuss going long periods without shampooing your hair. The scalp is a part of your skin, so it requires attention in terms of cleansing. The hair needs to be shampooed every 7 to 14 days and if one has locks then 21 days at the max but 3 to 4 weeks is stretching it. Anything past 4-6 weeks you are entering the poor hygiene zone and I'm speaking as a person with locks. It's true that over curly hair doesn't produce as much oil as straight hair but over a period of time the hair does accumulate a certain amount of dirt and bacteria after weeks without being shampooed. If the hair is locked, it no longer sheds because all of that hair is matted together to form the lock. With that in mind, you must be conscious of everything the hair holds over long periods of time and by long periods of time I mean weeks without cleansing. Dirt, oil, product buildup, smoke, fried food smells, germs, bacteria and even dead insects, if you are not careful, can all be festering within a head of locks that are not cleansed properly or at all for that matter. If every time you pass someone, you leave an odor behind from your hair, then you may need to do something about it. Bottom line, going long periods of time without shampooing the hair is a poor hygiene practice.

Are you looking for a hairstylist or a babysitter....
" I know the website has all the information I need, but can you hold my hand and walk me through it anyway?"

One of the simplest things we can do to avoid confusion is to research, read and pay attention. I can't elaborate on this section without sounding like a condescending smart ass soooo........moving on!
Disclaimer: This excludes older generations and those that are technologically challenged.

Leave it to the professionals..."My hair is a hot ghetto mess, but excuse the interrogation"

If your hair is damaged from what you've been doing to it or have allowed someone else to do to it, please don't question the stylist to death with a bunch of social media questions about whether organic or sulfate free products are used. If the stylist is licensed, they have access to professional products at the beauty supply store for licensed professionals. Research on the person touching you, products and techniques used needed to be done before you got to such a damaged state. So, allow your stylist to do their job without interference. A good stylist can tell by looking at your hair what's been done to it and will use the products necessary to bring the hair back to a healthy state. Of course, this will not be done in one appointment and yes, I must add that because some clients come in like they've been in a dog fight (that they've lost) and expect nothing more than a miracle before they leave the salon. Keep expectations realistic and leave it to the professionals. For the record, everyone with a license isn't a professional, they just happened to pass state board. Unfortunately, the industry is suffering from "boot leg kitchen beautician" syndrome and they're everywhere like some kind of bad virus. They're in their bathrooms on the internet or in salons full of state board violations..... so buyer beware!

Contrary to popular belief, we have a life.... What part of "I'm not your slave" don't you understand?

I know it's hard to accept that your stylist has things to do outside of the salon other than your hair, but it happens. Therefore, every occasionally, the answer will be no to a hair request and what's with not respecting the work space?! This does NOT apply to my clients because they have manners, but I've had the misfortune to work on some people who think they can parlay in the stylist's chairs, allow their children to run around the salon like it's a playground then have the nerve to try and get insulted because the unruly children didn't get serviced by who they thought should do them. The title stylist does not include a tail although some people treat their pets better than humans. Last time I looked, there was a butt back there and not a tail. Ok next!

Chapter Two

Hair Textures and Curl Patterns

There seems to be some confusion about the difference between hair textures and curl patterns. In the past and believe it or not in current day, people still think that a tight curl pattern means coarse and now hair is described in numbers and letters to further confuse women about their hair. This will allow some people to avoid hearing the word coarse to describe their hair and you know how Blacks folks hate that description which doesn't apply to a lot of tightly coiled curly hair types in terms of texture. Coarse, by the way is not a bad thing and for the most part straight hair or wavy hair can have a coarse texture. Hair texture represents how the hair feels and can be described as follows:

1. **Fine** - this is hair that is soft to the touch and easily damaged and usually missing the medulla which is the inner most section of the hair shaft.
2. **medium** - this hair type tends to be easier to manage and can take more heat than fine hair but not as wiry as coarse hair.
3. **Coarse** - this hair type tends to be very wiry and if the hair is straight it's difficult to curl and if the hair is curly it's difficult to straighten. Coarse hair does not mean bad nor does it describe a particular ethnic group's hair. It only describes how the hair feels.

A head of hair can also have different textures and curl patterns in different areas of the head. The top potion of the hair is usually straighter than the rest of the hair. The sides and back are usually curlier and thicker and the middle top portion usually has a texture that's a little more wirery than the rest of the hair. The temple area does not have a lot of pores so there's less hair in that area, but it doesn't mean a person is going bald.

Curl Patterns
This describes the direction in which the hair curls or doesn't curl as is the case with straight hair and goes as follows:
Keep in mind that the photos below are mere examples of basic curl patterns and there can be a combination of curl patterns on one head of hair that is not shown in a photo.

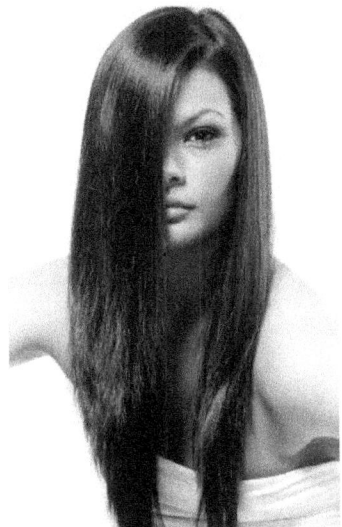

Straight

Wavy

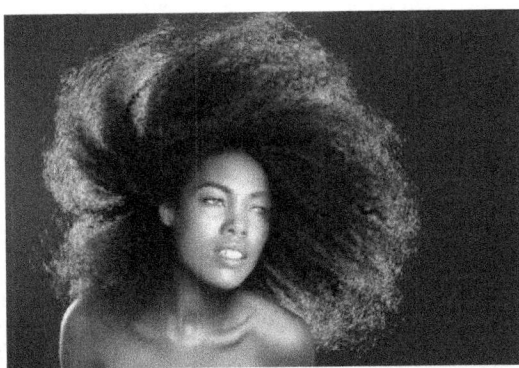

Curly

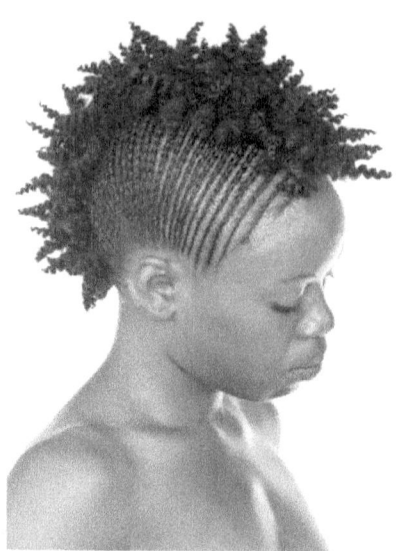

Over Curly or Kinky

Structure of The Hair

Here we have the "yawn" section and even though it may not be all that interesting, I feel it's important to know how the hair grows. We are so concerned with the hair shaft once it grows out of the scalp (which is biologically dead when it grows past the epidermis layer) when we need to be more concerned about the root, the bulb and the papilla because this is where the blood flows. If the blood doesn't flow to these areas then the hair doesn't grow, it's that simple.

HAIR ANATOMY

Hair shaft - is made of dead protein cells called keratin which is why there is no pain when the hair is cut. The main function of the hair is to protect the head.

Scalp - is made of soft tissue that covers the skull and has the same structure as skin.

Sebaceous Gland - an oil producing gland found beneath the scalp attached to hair follicles.

Hair Papilla - a knoblike indentation at the bottom of the hair follicle which is where the hair bulb fits.

Hair Erector Muscle - a muscle connected to the hair follicle and skin that responds to temperatures causing the hair to be erect or goose bumps on the skin.

Hair Follicle - a structure in the skin from which the hair grows.

Hair Root - part of the hair embedded in the hair follicle.

Hair Bulb - where living cells divide and grow to build the hair shaft.

Blood Vessel -tubular structure in which blood circulates.

Medulla - usually found in thick or coarse hair and is not found in naturally blonde and/or fine hair.

Cortex – middle layer that determines the strength, elasticity, and texture of the hair. Changes in the structure of the hair such as wet styling, thermal styling, coloring, perming or relaxing takes place in the cortex. Contains melanin which gives the hair it color.

Cuticle – contains overlapping scale-like cells that gives the hair shaft its strength and prevents damage to the inner structure of the hair.

Growth Phases

There are times when clients often complain about hair loss not realizing they are experiencing a phase of shedding. Hair grows during different phases on different parts of the head to prevent shedding all at once. Below is an example of the hair's growth cycle.

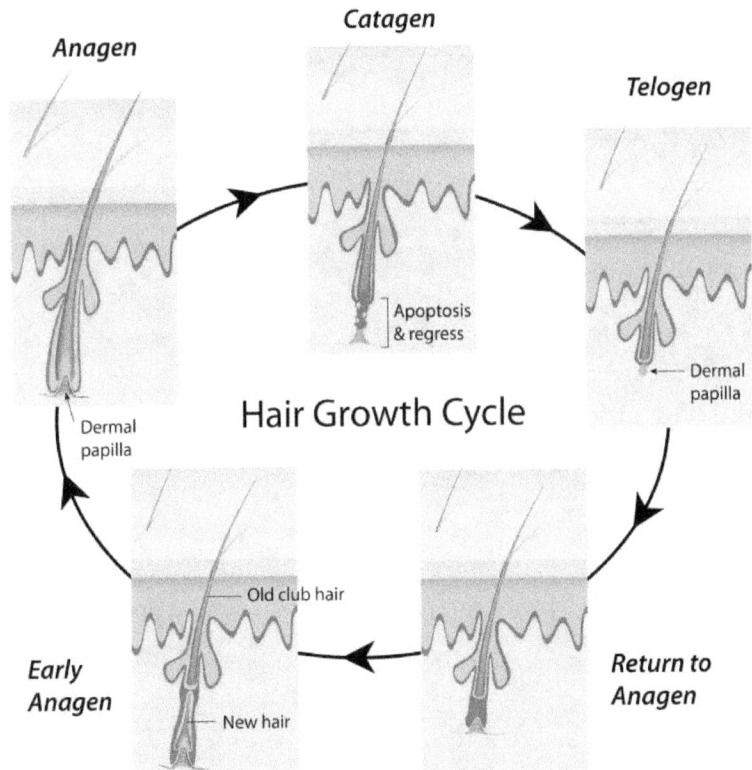

Anagen - growth phase (cells in the papilla or root divide to produce new hair). About 85% of the hair is in this phase at one time producing hair that grows thick.

Catagen - transitional or regression phase is the time when the hair follicle renews itself. The hair follicle (root) shrinks and detaches (start to degenerate) from the dermal papilla and usually lasts about 10 days. Apoptosis or cell death happens during this phase

Telogen – resting phase which is the result of normal hair loss called shedding. The resting phase lasts about three months with 10-15% of the hair in this phase. New hair begin the early anagen phase while the old hair is resting.

Early Anagen - Old hair falls out to make room for new hair growing in.

Chapter Three

Types of Hair Loss

Keep in mind that all hair loss is alopecia but there different types. Here are some of the types below.

Traction Alopecia – Caused by damage done to the papilla and hair follicle from constant pulling or tension over a long period of time from hair styles such as braids, cornrows, and ponytails.

Androgenic Alopecia – Genetically determined disorder commonly found in men and women know has pattern baldness.

Alopecia Areata – An auto immune skin condition where the immune system mistakenly attacks hair follicles causing a disruption in the hair's growth cycle preventing the hair from growing above the skin's surface.

Anagen Effluvium – Hair shedding and thinning that occur during the growth phase of the hair life cycle as a result of exposure to chemicals or toxins (chemotherapy or radiation).

Telogen Effluvium – Shedding and thinning caused by stress or illness.

Central centrifugal cicatricial alopecia – CCCA naturally occurs as a result of tight hairstyles or chemical burns from perms and relaxers. Most common in African American women. Also known as scarring alopecia.

Hair Loss Contributors

Medication – chemotherapy/radiation, high blood pressure medication, epidural.
Illness – Lupus (autoimmune disease where healthy body tissue is attacked by its own immune system), anemia (blood deficiency), ringworm (fungal infection that cause hair to break once it is in the hair fibers).

Menopause - (when a woman's period stops and she can no longer get pregnant). Hair loss is temporary.

Giving birth - (the rise in hormones keeps the hair from falling out and once the hair returns to normal, hair loss occurs usually within 3 months).

Psychological Conditions Trichotillomania – self- induced hair loss as a result of continuous pulling on the hair.

Stress – All hair loss is stressful, but some conditions can directly contribute to hair loss such as major surgery, child birth, crash diets that do not contain enough protein, high fever or severe infection, birth control pills and some anti - depressants, toxic relationships and an unhealthy mate. That's right, an unhealthy mate because whatever he puts into his body, he puts into you during intercourse. If he's emotionally unhealthy, then those negative emotions are transferred to you also. I emphasize the effect on the female because women take in while the male puts out. In all fairness, men should be mindful of an emotionally negative woman also because stress is a killer!

Resting Phase – hair growth stops and sheds then is replaced by new hair during the beginning of the Anagen phase.

Skin and Scalp Disorders

Scalp disorders are no fun and can be frustrating when everything you try doesn't work, but here are some examples of skin and scalp disorders to be aware of.

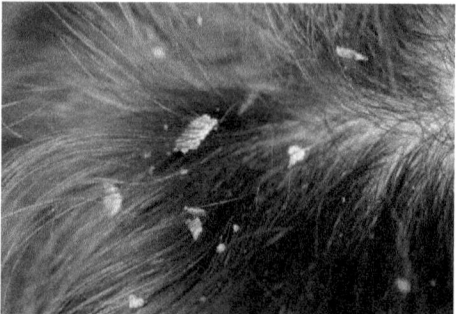

Dandruff – symptoms include flaky scalp that may or may not itch and is pastier than dry scalp. It can be caused by a sensitivity to yeast, fungal infection (a fungus feeding off of the oils the hair follicle secretes will grow out if control and cause the scalp to become irritated and produce extra skin cells), poor circulation to the scalp, a diet deficient in zinc and B vitamins, or the use of high alkaline shampoo and hair products.

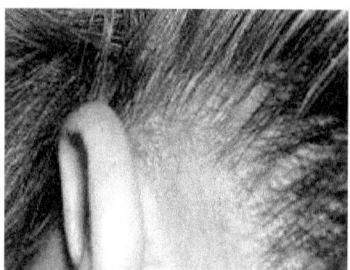

Seborrheic Dermatitis – Is similar to dandruff but involves more of an inflammation of the scalp along with burning and itching,

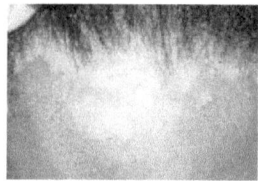

Eczema – symptoms include itching, skin inflammation, red patches, dry thickened skin and or tiny blisters and are associated with asthma, an allergic type reaction of the body, food allergies, dysfunctional immune system, low stomach acid, or stress.

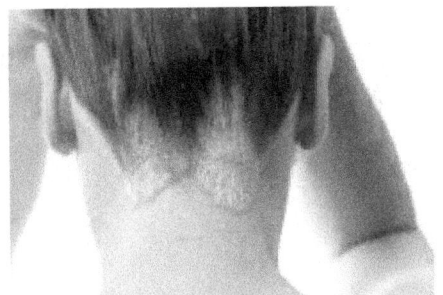

Psoriasis – when the body makes too many skin cells leaving an excess of skin cells on the scalp.

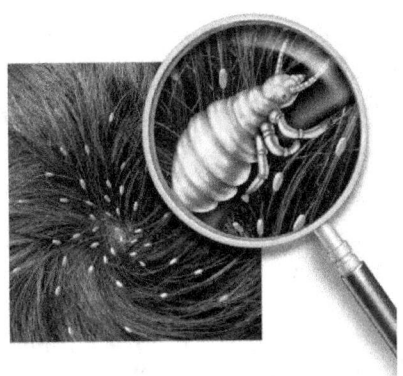

Lice – An insect that feeds off the host's blood supply and the female lays eggs on the hair shaft. According to what the books in cosmetology describe, lice do not survive in over curly hair because it suffocates. Also, heat styling and chemical styling prevent lice from latching on to the hair. Being from a particular race doesn't make one immune from lice, but whether or not the hair provides an environment for the lice to survive depends on the texture and curl pattern of the hair.

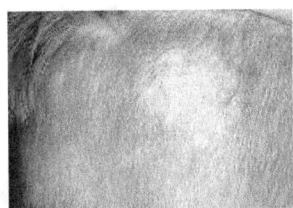

Ringworm – A fungal infection leaving ring like rashes resulting in hair loss.

Diet and Nutrition

The number one question I get concerning hair is, "What product do you recommend for my hair?" We are constantly looking for the quick topical fix when the answer lies in what we put into our bodies whether its food, vitamin supplements, cell food or plain old fashioned water.

Supplements:

Beta Carotene – an antioxidant the body turns into vitamin A which produces oils that sustain the scalp. People low in vitamin A usually have dandruff. Other foods with beta carotene include orange and yellow vegetables like carrots and squash, tomato products and fruits such as cantaloupe.

Biotin – improves the keratin infrastructure of the hair, recommended dosage 2.5 mg.; signs of overdose: lower vitamin c and b6 levels, skin rashes, and slow release of insulin, high blood sugar levels. Other foods with biotin include cereal, eggs, milk, legumes and chocolate.

Iron – transmits oxygen to the hair follicles helping the body use protein to grow and build strong hair. Iron deficiency will result in anemia. Other foods with iron include red meat, dark leafy green vegetables and dried fruits such as prunes and raisins.

Omega 3 – polyunsaturated (found in plant-based foods and oils) fatty acids adds luster sheen and elasticity preventing the hair from being dry and brittle therefore reducing hair loss. Other foods with omega 3 include anchovies, tuna, mackerel and sardines.

Protein – are large molecules that consist of amino acids which the body and the cells in the body need to function properly. 90% of the hair is made of protein therefore the hair needs protein to grow. A lack of protein can lead to poor immune function, lack of energy and muscle weakness. Other foods with protein include beans and lean poultry.

Vitamin C – an antioxidant that aids in the circulation to the scalp and supports tiny blood vessels that feed the follicles. Other foods with vitamin c include citrus fruits like oranges, cantaloupe, mango, papaya, vegetables such as chili peppers, red and green bell peppers, kale and broccoli.

Vitamin E – in topical form, it increases blood flow to the scalp promoting faster growth and thickness. Also great for the skin. Green leafy vegetables such as Parsley, Spinach, Kale, and Broccoli contain vitamin E.

Zinc – a mineral that helps the body repair and grow hair; keeps the oil glands of the hair working properly. Also aids in preventing hair loss. Other foods include beef, lamb, sesame seeds and pumpkin seeds.

Chapter Four

Products and Their Use

One of the most common issues I face with new clients, is an overuse of product on the hair or not using the correct product for their hair type or skin and scalp condition. Clients, before taking on a regular hair maintenance routine, usually over condition their hair which will cause the hair to be too soft and become gummy or they'll over moisturize the hair with oils or a cream hair dress which will cause the hair to actually be drier once it is shampooed. The dryness occurs when the hair is stripped of all oil and dirt by the sulfate shampoo and the hair is not allowed to produce its own oils to moisturize the hair because it has been weighed down with oil-based products. Clients tend to think using a sulfate shampoo will dry the hair out (and it will if over used) when in fact using the sulfate free shampoo, based on my experience, will not always properly cleanse the hair of oil and dirt. Sulfate shampoos contain ingredients that will draw oil and dirt, once it is combined with water, in order to clean the hair. Remember that products are to maintain the hair and hydrating the body along with a healthy diet will greatly contribute to a head of healthy hair.

Below, I've listed some common scalp issues and recommendations for the type of product containing ingredients that can be used for that issue.

Issue/Ingredient:

Dry Scalp/Dandruff – coal tar (natural anti-fungal agent), tea tree (anti-fungal, antiseptic, antibiotic), ketoconazole (kills the yeast or fungus that cause dandruff), selenium sulfide (kills yeast and reduces the scalps cell regeneration speed).

Thin Hair – Ingredients such as keratin protein in volumizing products coat the cuticle of the hair causing it to expand giving the illusion of thicker fuller hair.

Dry Hair – sulfate-free shampoos containing sodium lauroyl methyl isethionate are good for moisturizing the hair.

Product build up – Here's where sulfate shampoos are necessary because they break up oil and dirt and remove it from the hair. Of course too much of anything is bad for you and over use of cleansers will cause dryness and irritation so use in moderation. For those experiencing allergic reactions, vinegar based shampoo will remove product build up.

Grey Hair – purple shampoos rid grey hair of yellow and keep it white. Purple is the opposite of yellow on the color wheel cancelling out the yellow.

Chemically treated - thermal products protect the hair from heat styling while adding moisture and shine to the hair

Color Treated - These products are designed to keep color vibrant after shampooing.

Tools

Trying to figure out what product to use seems to be the main focus of a lot of people when it comes to their hair, but choosing the right tools is just as important as proper product use. Here are a few examples of the types of tools you should use according to the style you are trying to create.

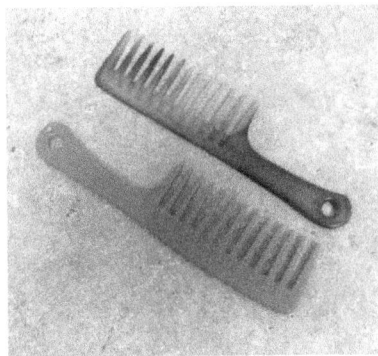

Large tooth comb - this type of comb is great for combing the hair while wet with the use of conditioner to aid in detangling the hair.

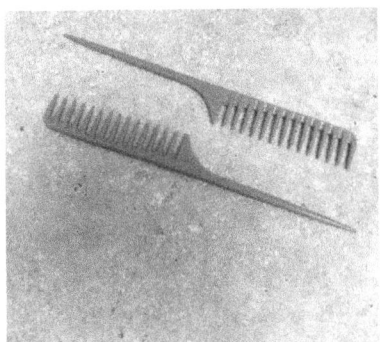

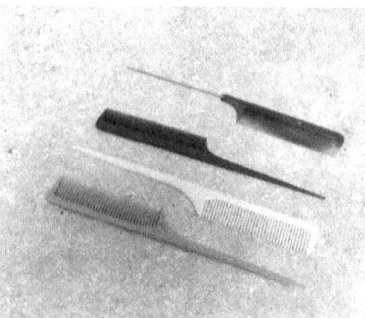

Rattail comb - use this type of comb to part the hair or assist when doing straight styles. Rattail combs are not to be used to comb out the hair; a large tooth comb should always be used for this purpose.

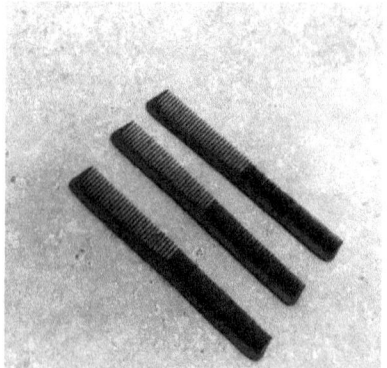

Styling comb/cutting comb - these combs are specifically for controlling the hair while it is being cut or trimmed.

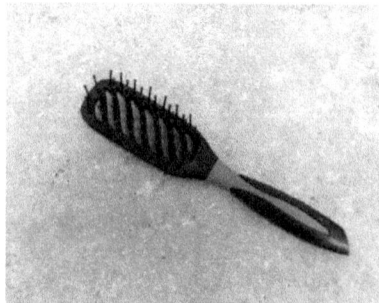

Vent brush - use this brush with the rubber tips to de-tangle the hair when taking out braids, weaves or brushing through the hair while it is wet with conditioner. It can get through the hair much easier than a comb when the hair is tangled.

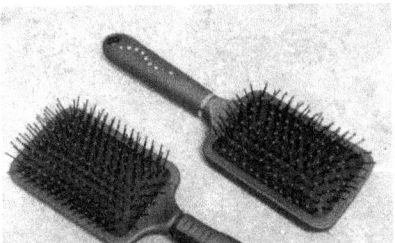

Paddle brush - use this brush to help straighten the hair while it is being blow-dried.

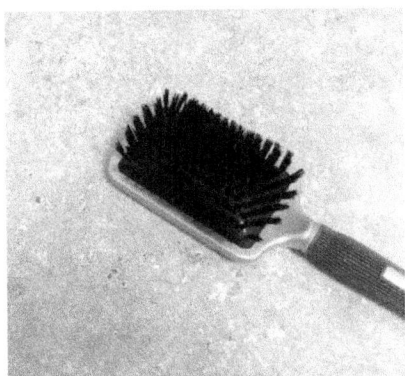

Boar bristle brush - this is the brush to use when the hair is worn in a straight style and is going to be wrapped to preserve the hair style. The fiber in the boar bristle will be much more gentle on the hair than a brush made of plastic.

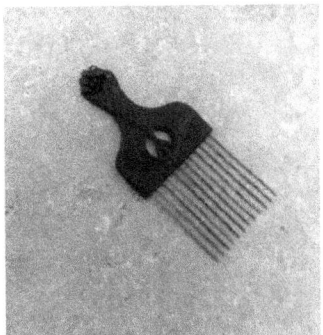

Afro pick - pretty much the name speaks for itself because this is the best tool to use if you are wearing an Afro because it will enable you to pick out the hair evenly in order to maintain a neat style.

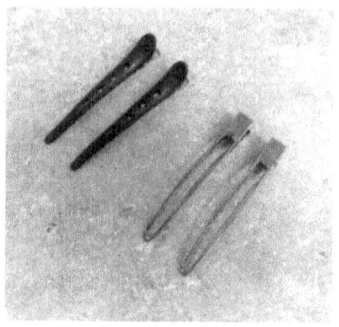

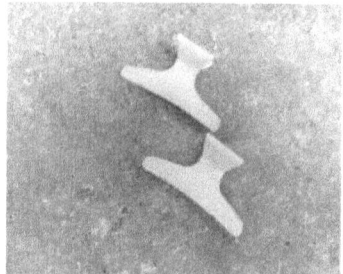

Clips - these items are used to control the hair and keep it out of the way while styling or blow drying.

Flexi Rods, Spiral Rods, Perm Rods - Used to create spiral curls

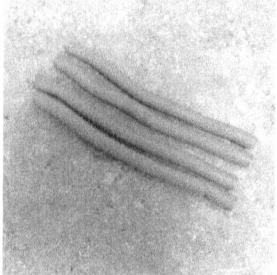

Flexi Rods

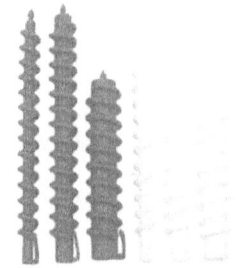

Spiral Rods

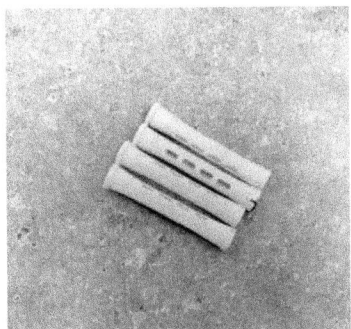

Perm Rods

Hair Maintenance Techniques

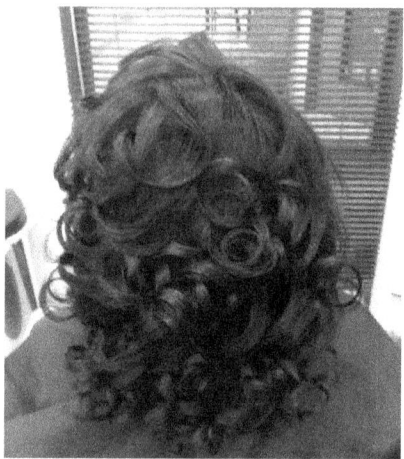

Photo by JW Salon Styles

Shampoo and Style on Chemical Free Hair

Tools Needed:

Shampoo, conditioner, hot oil if necessary, thermal protectant, cream moisturizer, oil sheen or glossifier, paddle brush, rat tail comb, clips and blow dryer.

Step 1.

Shampoo the hair using a cleansing shampoo to remove oil and dirt following up with a second or third shampoo depending on the needs of the hair that is designed for thermal styling.

Step 2.

Apply conditioner (thermal product) to the hair and hot oil on the scalp (hot oil is optional) and place under the dryer with plastic cap for 10-15 minutes. Sitting under the dryer will aid in the flat ironing process allowing the straightening to last longer.

Step 3.

Rinse thoroughly with luke warm to cool water, towel dry then spray the hair with thermal protectant.

Step 4.

Section the hair for control and begin blow drying starting at the nape area and work towards the front of the hair using the paddle brush or comb attachment if you're doing it yourself.

Step 5.
Apply moisturizer, hair dress or serum prior to using the flat iron before straightening the hair particularly around the perimeter of the head. Moisturizer may be omitted when straightening fine hair and a glossifier can be used as a substitute.

Step 6.
After straightening the edges, start at the nape area taking small sections and flat iron the hair until the process is complete.

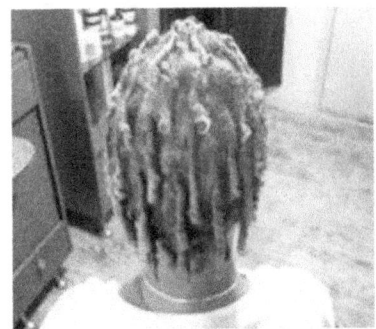

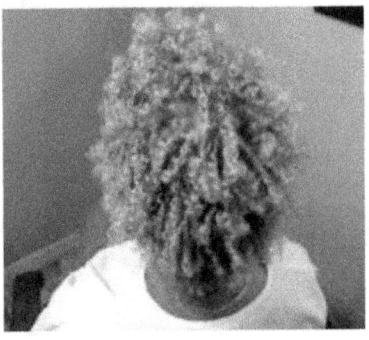

Photos by JW Salon Styles

Twist Out Using Comb Twists:

Tools Needed:
Shampoo, conditioner, product to twist, setting lotion, comb, clips, gel glossifier.

Step 1.

Shampoo the hair to remove oil and dirt using a cleansing shampoo then follow up with a sulphate free shampoo to soften.

Step 2.
Apply a detangling conditioner, comb through and rinse. Sitting under the dryer not necessary.

Step 3.
Starting at the nape area, use the comb to twist the hair in a coil and continue through to the front of the head until the process is complete.

Step 4.
Place under the dryer for 50-60 minutes until the hair is dry.

Step 5.
After drying, take each twist and make smaller twists using your fingers and the gel glossifier to coil the hair clock wise until all of the hair is done.

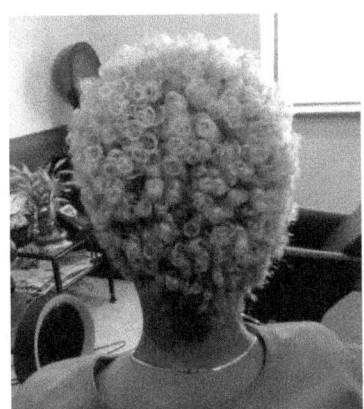
Photo by JW Salon Styles

Twist Out Using Flexi Rods

Tools Needed:
Shampoo, detangling conditioner, setting lotion, product to rod the hair, comb, clips, gel glossifier.

Step 1.
Shampoo the hair to remove oil and dirt with a cleansing shampoo then follow up with a sulphate free shampoo to soften.

Step 2.
Apply detangling conditioner, comb through and rinse.

Step 3.
Apply setting lotion and/or foam wrap product to rod the hair.

Step 4.
Starting at the nape area, begin to rod the hair in a spiral motion along the length of the rod then secure it by folding it together. Continue this process until the entire head is done.

Step 5.
Place under the dryer for 50-60 minutes until the hair is dry.

Step 6.
After drying, remove the rods by carefully unwrapping the hair and re-curling it back in place with your fingers.

Step 7.
Using the gel glossifier, divide the hair into smaller curls twisting clock wise until all of the hair is separated.

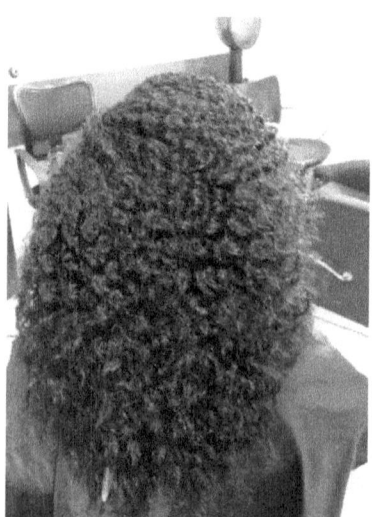

Photo by JW Salon Styles

Twist Out Using Flat Twist

Tools Needed:
Shampoo, detangling conditioner, setting lotion, product to twist, rat tail comb, wide tooth comb, clips, gel glossifier.

Step 1.
Shampoo hair to remove oil and dirt.

Step 2.
Apply detangling conditioner, comb through and rinse.

Step 3.
Apply setting lotion and product to twist.

Step 4.
Section the hair as if doing cornrows and begin flat twisting the hair starting at the front of the head working back to the nape area. Continue this process until the head is done.

Step 5.
Place under the dryer for 50-60 minutes but this style turns out better with overnight drying.

Step 6.
Using the gel glossifier, apply it to the hair to untwist it. Fluff it out and the style is complete.

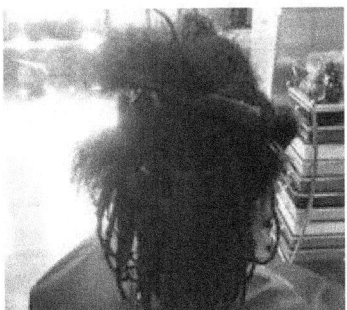

Yarn Added Photo by JW Salon Styles

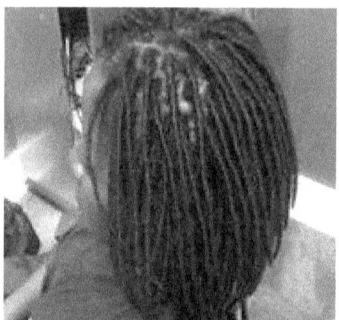

Afro Kinky Hair Wrapped
Photo by JW Salon Styles

Loc Extension

Tools Needed:
Shampoo, leave in conditioner, blow dryer, rat tail comb, wide tooth comb, clips, yarn, afro kinky hair, bonding glue (optional).

Step 1.
Shampoo the hair to remove oil and dirt

Step 2.
Apply a small amount of leave in to manage the hair while combing.

Step 3.
Blow dry the hair to remove moisture and section before braiding.

Step 4.
Starting at the nape, take sections according to the size of loc desired (one piece of yarn for small locs, two pieces for medium locs and three for and braid or twist the yarn in to the hair.

Step 5.
Apply bonding glue (if using) along the yarn braid and wrap it with the afro kinky hair. Palm roll it to smooth and secure the hair on the braid. Continue this process until the whole head is done. Takes 9-12 hours depending on size started.

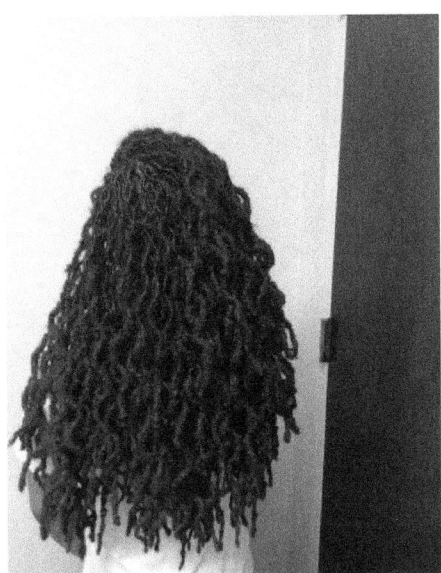
Photo by J W Salon Styles

Loc Maintenance

Tools Needed:
Shampoo, leave in conditioner, scalp oil, product to twist, clips, oil sheen or liquid glossifier.

Step 1.
Shampoo the hair to remove oil and dirt.

Step 2.
Apply leave in conditioner to the hair and oil to the scalp.

Step 3.
Apply product for twisting to the new growth throughout the hair.

Step 4.
Starting at the nape area, palm roll each loc clockwise and secure with a clip. Continue this process until all of the hair is twisted.

Step 5.
Place under the dryer 15 minutes if styling or 30-40 minutes without styling.

Step 6.
Spray with oil sheen and complete the finished look with a style.

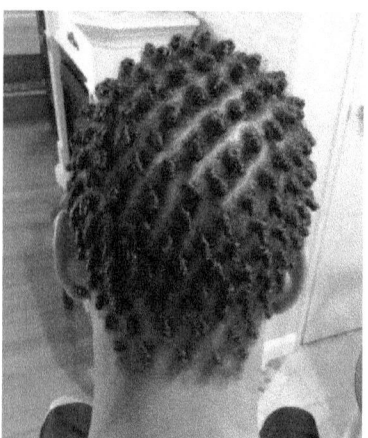
Photo by JW Salon Styles

Starting Locs With Comb Twists

Tools Needed:
Shampoo, leave in conditioner, large tooth comb to detangle, small tooth comb to twist, clips, setting lotion, product to twist, oil sheen or glossifier.

Step 1.
Shampoo the hair with a cleansing shampoo to remove oil and dirt.

Step 2.
Apply leave in conditioner to the hair for manageability while combing

Step 3.
Spray setting lotion and apply product for twisting

Step 4.
Section the hair according to the size of loc desired keeping in mind that the size you start will swell during the beginning phase and shrink done in size as the loc matures.

Step 5.
Continue this process until the whole head is complete.

Step 6.
Place under the dryer for 50-60 minutes until the hair is dry and spray with glossifier or oil sheen for shine to complete the style. The hair should be re-twisted every two weeks until the hair mats enough to be palm rolled.

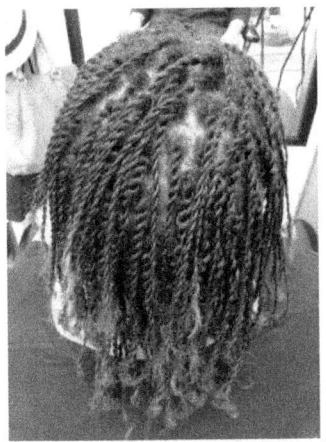

Two strand twist without style
Photo by JW Salon Styles

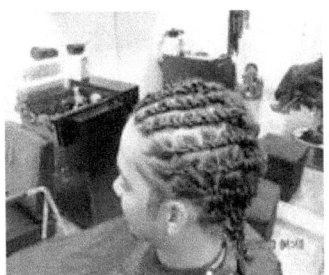

Two strand twist with style to start locs
Photo by JW Salon Styles

Starting Locs With Two Strand Twists

Tools Needed:
Shampoo, leave in conditioner, large tooth comb for detangling, rat tail comb, clips, product to twist.

Step 1.
Shampoo hair to remove oil and dirt.

Step 2.
Apply leave in conditioner and comb through.

Step 3.
Section hair beginning at the nape area according to the size of loc desired keeping in mind that each two strand will be two locs once they are separated.

Step 4.
In a twist and roll motion cross the two sections of hair of each other to form a small rope and continue this process until the whole head is twisted.

Step 5.
Style hair in an up do to keep it neat and re- twist every two weeks until the hair is ready to be palm rolled.

Loc Phases:

1-3 months - the hair is smooth and begins to mat and swell a bit, but is still soft enough to come apart when the hair is shampooed. Depending on texture, curl pattern and length, palm rolling can began by the third month. I personally prefer to style as soon as possible so the hair stays tight until the clients next appointment. It also speeds up the locking process.

3-6 months - the hair starts matting more, starting from the ends, working its way up closer to the scalp. There may be a little bit of hair that separates from the ends, but that's normal and nothing to be concerned about. Due to an extreme case of the "fuzzies", the hair will be in an in between stage where it looks almost locked but not. Hair is usually palm rolled or twisted by this time.

6-9 months - oh that shrinkage! Just when you thought you're getting some length, the hair starts to shrink and that's because the matting process is allowing the loc to become firmer and a little more solid. For some, depending on the texture and curl pattern, you're still going through the first two phases so keep in mind the process isn't the same for everyone.

9-12 months - Ok so you're finally on your way to a beautiful locked look (or at least you should be), but if not hang tight and continue with maintenance and it will be worth it in the end. The locs are tighter and less puffy than in previous months and have taken on a neater appearance.

12-18 months - Locs are more solid and longer of course. The size that is started should be a bit smaller than the size you hope to achieve because the hair is no longer shedding like loose hair that is being combed and will eventually increase in size before it tightens after maturity. Also, if the textured is fine, I recommend starting small anyway to prevent breakage when the locs mature and become long. Smaller locs are not as heavy and have more flexibility with styling.

Maintenance According To Hair Style

The following product types are just suggestions and not necessarily items that have to be used for these styles. I do not endorse any particular product line, but the glossary will provide you with product ingredients to look for when choosing a hair care line.

Twist outs –It's amazing what a few techniques can do to change the outcome of a hairstyle. Years ago we didn't have a clue as to how to obtain a curly look without using rollers, a curling iron, or adding hair. Now with a few different tools and again some different techniques women can achieve hairstyles that can be worn for a least two weeks and not have to worry about sweating because the style actually looks better as it gets a little older. I pride myself on having almost every hairstyle, but since I've had locs, I haven't had the experience of wearing a twist out with the flexi rods just two strand. Most of the products that would be used for this hairstyle is applied while the style is being created therefore maintenance is minimal for the client. Products such as scalp oil, spray glossifiers, or oil sheen would suffice in maintaining the style until it is redone. Products used to create the style usually have a cream consistency with oils and other ingredients that moisturize the hair. Setting lotion or wrap foam locks the style in place during the twisting process. I don't recommend a gel product because the hair will harden once it is dried and could possibly cause flaking.

Afros - Again the goal is to moisturize so use a cream product such as a hair dress for the hair and oil for the scalp. It's also important to keep the ends clean with a trim or hair cut so the style will be shaped properly and use oil sheen to add shine to the finished look.

Locs – These products are usually oil based or water based and applied while the hair is wet in order for the hair to be twisted properly. If a product causes a buildup or flakes in the hair, discontinue use. At this point, removal of product buildup will happen over a period of time after a series of shampoos. Again, going a long time without shampooing the hair can cause buildup in the hair from dry scalp or even lint.

Chemical Free – Products for heat styling include thermal protectant (which seals the cuticle and protects the hair from heat damage) for blow drying, hair dress (for moisturizing) or glossifier (adds shine without oil) for styling and oil sheen for the finished looked.

Braids and Cornrows – It's best to use oils on the scalp that will penetrate and hydrate the hair while it is braided. Remember not to allow your hair to be braided too tightly because the scalp naturally swells from the tension. If braids are tight from the beginning then the process of traction alopecia will begin. You see it when the hair around the edges have the white bulb on the tip. The hair is coming out from the root at this point.

Weaves – You don't want to put too much product on the scalp with weaves or extensions because it can make the hair that is added oily and after a couple of weeks the hair will smell. Shampooing every two weeks is highly recommended and applying a glossifier or oil sheen is all that is needed for maintenance. The key to keeping your hair healthy while wearing a weave is to remove it within the 6 to 8 week period, have it shampooed, treated, conditioned, and trimmed before putting in new extensions. If these steps are done regularly the hair will stay intact. If the weave is worn past its 6 to 8 weeks, damage is done to the new growth. The hair will mildew or dry rot from being wet and not properly dried or damaged from being re-stitched during tightening. As a professional I don't recommend tightening for weaves because it damages the hair underneath. If you need tightening, then it's probably time to take it out especially if you want to protect your edges.

Chapter Five

Real Talk

Here's the part where I say things I'm probably not supposed to say because it would be offensive or shocking to those who may be guilty of some of the behavior I want to speak on. The natural hair care evolution is a wonderful thing and finally women of color are embracing their natural hair that grows out of their head and are not hiding behind an identity that's not their own. When we chemically alter our curl pattern or straighten it with heat, it damages the hair but I am not condemning those who choose to continue with this process because I was once there and people have to do what feels comfortable for them. I've seen quite a few women who were attempting to wear their hair in its natural state and it just wasn't working for them. They were uncomfortable with how they looked and their attempts at styles were less than successful.

Terminology

Before I go into that topic allow me to begin by speaking on terminology as it relates to ethnic hair. As professionals we don't use the term white hair or black hair because there are people of color with straight hair such as the Aborigines (although some have curly hair too) which are the Black Australians, Native American, just to name a few. These are darker people with straight hair and then you have those that would be considered Anglo such as some Italians and some people from Spain as well as some Asian people (Indian, Korean, Thai, etc.) who have curly or over curly curl patterns. Wavy, curly, over curly or kinky hair is just not limited to the American African or African person. So it is important not to label hair according to race because that would be considered improper terminology. Curl patterns are not to be confused with hair texture as I explained before in previous chapters; curl patterns describe the direction the hair grows and textures represent how the hair feels.

One more thing......stop calling relaxers perms!!!!! Relaxers, containing sodium hydroxide lye or calcium hydroxide lye, straighten the hair and perms containing calcium, sodium, potassium or ammonium thioglycolate curl the hair. During the age of the conks in the early 20's, the only term available to us was perm which was used to curl straight hair on Caucasians and for some reason, we've continued to use the term to describe hair straighteners even though it says relaxer on the product. Old habits are hard to break I guess.

Straight hair attitude versus natural hair attitude

Some of you may have noticed this and some of you may not have noticed, hell maybe some of you are just in denial of this mere observation. This doesn't pertain to all women that relax their hair and wear weaves or extensions but from my personal observation, I've noticed that there is more drama, tension, and conflict amongst women who straighten and or wear fake hair (and what's with the hostility?). I had to examine my own attitude and thought process when I was wearing a weave and getting my hair relaxed. A room full of these women is full of gossip, backbiting and women just hating on other females about superficial bull shit like shoes, clothes and how good or bad someone else's hair looks. Whereas a room with sistahs that are natural have a totally different vibe. I mean it's practically drama free and much more complementary. The women have a confidence that women who chemically alter their hair or where extensions just don't have and it's the truth based on what I've observed in the beauty profession over 25 plus years. When my hair was relaxed or weaved I was constantly aware of my hair and it occupied a large portion of my thoughts throughout the day and I didn't have the best attitude either. I felt the reason why so many black women didn't get along was because they hated themselves and if they saw any part of themselves that they hated in another woman then there would be conflict. I feel it's more subconscious than conscience and again this doesn't apply to all women because there are some women out there with natural hair and synthetic minds and they don't always know how to act either so...... next topic.

Poor hygiene is a disease you don't want to catch (yeah here it is again)

Newsflash people, going long periods without shampooing your hair is poor hygiene because the scalp is a part of your body and requires cleansing every 7 to 14 days and MAYBE a little longer if you are locked but for some reason there are people who think it's okay to wear a style past its cleansing time or point simply because it doesn't look bad. SHAMPOO YOUR DAMN HAIR!!!!! There are germs and bacteria crawling all through the hair and scalp which can cause skin and scalp issues such as an overabundance of cell production as in the case of dandruff which by the way is not normal or necessarily hereditary and can be controlled through diet, regular waste elimination from the body, and cleansing on a regular basis. Also, clean and sanitize combs and brushes to prevent scalp issues.

Acne can occur when the skin around the forehead and temple area is not cleansed properly and oil and dirt from the hair coupled with what's floating around in the elements sits on the skin. Hair loss or alopecia can result from many things and not just a lack of shampooing the hair. For example, wearing braids or weaves for 1 to 2 months or more without shampooing the hair. The lack of shampooing, the traction from the tension the style creates and the product buildup in accumulation with oil and dirt are all contributing factors to potential damage done to the scalp and hair.

And WHAT THE F%#K IS A CO-WASH?!!! I'll tell you what it is; it's a ho bath for the hair and personally, I don't understand why people are doing the "hot spot" wash on their hair. Oh, you know what the hot spot wash is; under arms, between your legs and the crack of your be-hind! Co washing is cleansing the hair with conditioner instead of shampoo, but if conditioner were meant for cleansing, it would be in the shampoo section.

Even if the conditioner contains a small amount of surfactants which are detergents, it isn't enough to properly cleanse the hair. Sodium lauryl sulfate is not your enemy but merely a detergent whose job is to pull oil and dirt away from the hair when combined with water to cleanse and of course it will dry the hair out if over used or used improperly. A sulfate free shampoo should follow a sulfate shampoo after the hair has been stripped of oil (from products) and dirt and is squeaky clean. The sulfate free shampoo then softens the hair after it has been cleansed. If your hair doesn't have any product build up that needs to be removed then by all means use other cleansers that are sulfate free, but remember to choose the product according to your specific hair care situation. If you're allergic to sodium lauryl sulfate, you'll find what ingredient to look for in a sulfate free shampoo in the glossary section.

The Quick Fix…..Putting a band aid on an open wound doesn't work either

The quick fix is something we are all guilty of wanting, but it usually doesn't work out for the best because you will eventually find yourself right back where you started. As it relates to hair, the quick fix is hair products applied to hair that need so much more than topical treatments. Maintenance products are designed to maintain something that has already been going on such as a regular hair care routine. Yet women purchase endless amounts of product and use them as a cure all for hair growth, skin and scalp conditions and split ends. If it were that simple, everyone would have long healthy hair. All products don't work on everyone and a product should be chosen according to the hair type and hair issue if there is one.

It amazes me how some people don't relate what they put into their bodies with how it affects their hair and scalp. Proper hydration, steady blood flow from exercise, vitamin supplements, and healthy eating will contribute greatly to a head of strong shiny hair that is free of flakes.

Price according to skill level…..Please Read Carefully!

I feel the need to address this topic because for some reason some people think that prices should be the same everywhere when it comes to hair care services which doesn't make sense. So sorry to say, but it doesn't. Unfortunately there are those charging above their skill level as well as those charging below their skill level, but the terms student, junior stylist, intermediate stylist and master or senior stylist exist for a reason. The more advanced the skill level, the more one will pay for services. All cutting shears, flat irons, and blow dryers are not created equal and there is a reason why some tools cost more than others. Also, expect to pay more when making an appointment with someone with long term experience in the industry and a specialty service they provide. No one goes to the hospital and tell doctors how to perform surgery, but for some reason women and some men, who don't know any better, seem to think they can tell stylists how to do their job and all of a sudden almost everyone with no training can do hair. Anyone feeling the need to instruct a stylist should continue following the bootleg bathroom beauticians on the internet and do their own hair because we really don't need the headache. The client's only job is to convey WHAT they want and leave the HOW to the professional. There's more than one way to do things and just because the client may not be familiar with a technique, doesn't mean the style won't be complete.

Keeping The Hair You Have

1. **Shampoo the hair every 7-14 days** because anything longer than that technically would be considered "hygienically incorrect". In layman's terms, it just a poor hygiene practice although in the defense of some who have locs, more time usually goes by between shampoos. The scalp and hair may not produce the oil that straighter textures produce to attract dirt, but an accumulation of dirt and bacteria builds up on the scalp and hair shaft when the hair is not shampooed on a regular basis. This especially applies to locs since there is little to no hair that sheds from the head except on the ends. A person that wears locs can easily become nose blind to the smell that their hair emits and believe me, it stinks when it hasn't been shampooed. Locs will develop product build up combined with dirt and bacteria from the elements, work environments, food odors, and or smoke that settle on the hair and penetrate the loc. When this happens, it may take several shampoos to cleanse the loc thoroughly. You'll know your hair has a buildup when your hands or finger tips are sticky after shampooing the hair which is nothing more than old residue from accumulated oil and dirt.

2. **Get a trim** every 6-8 weeks to protect the hair from breakage. Contrary to misinformed popular belief, the hair grows out of the scalp and not from the ends so holding on to split ends doesn't maintain length. They're merely an illusion of length and should be cut immediately. Holding on to dead ends doesn't work for the hair because it causes more damage by splitting along the hair shaft which is why clients generally have to get a haircut when they finally go to a stylist. The hair grows every day except during the resting period of the telogen phase, but if the ends are split, as the hair grows from the scalp it breaks on the ends resulting in short or damaged hair. Let go of that which is no longer working for you.

3. **Be gentle with your hair** because it deserves your respect. A common issue I run across is shedding and excessive tangling due to rough handling while the hair is wet. The hair is at its weakest when it is wet. First shampoo the hair; using a vent brush or wide tooth comb, start detangling the hair from the ends and work your way up to the scalp after applying conditioner to the hair to soften it. Use the same technique after the conditioner is rinsed out and apply a spray or cream leave in conditioner or thermal spray or cream protectant before blow drying or styling.

Since when did giving a damn about how you looked become too much work?

During the natural/textured hair care explosion, I've noticed a rapid decline in the appearance of women. Some of you are taking the "I don't care" attitude about your image a little far. Would it be too much to ask that you complete your twist out before going in public? Where a hat or wrap until your hair is ready to come out of whatever is being done to set the hair. We live in a superficial society that judge us constantly by how we look and carry ourselves. Don't expect respect if you're looking like you don't care about or respect yourself. All I'm saying is maintain a neat appearance and care about your image when you leave the house because that's free. In defense of some free form looks, there are some beautiful afro styles, twist outs and locs out there that are clean, combed and shiny so these styles are NOT the ones I'm talking about. Throwing a head band on without combing your hair is a violation, mimicking hair styles on "water and lotion" hair girls when you have "power to the people" hair is a violation, denial is a waste of brain power so be realistic about what your hair can do and wear a style that fits you and your hair type. Oh and flakes on your clothes and in your eyebrows where other people can see it is a violation too. Just drink plenty of water and shampoo the hair and scalp with a product designed for scalp conditions.

It's not my intention to be harsh for my true intent is to inform and educate. When you know better you definitely do better. Take what you need and throw away the rest if you must but whether it be compliment or criticism, there's something to learn here. Happy hair days to everyone!

Do's and Don'ts

Do:

Cleanse the hair every 7-14 days: While working in Texas, I found the hair culture to be different than anything I've ever experienced in the hair care industry. Women would go one or more months without shampooing their hair and in their minds, if the style doesn't look bad, why get it redone. I don't know where this logic came from, but it is a bad hygiene practice and doesn't do the hair any good either. Every time we walk out into the elements, dust and germs attach to the hair not to mention we are shedding dead skin cells every day. In addition to this, some people have an overabundance of cell production (dandruff) because of their diet and or their inability to eliminate waste. Waiting such long periods to shampoo the hair only compounds the situation. One of the common complaints Black women have about their hair is dryness which can be caused by a lack a fluid intake, poor diet, no vitamin regimen, and product build up from the over use of oil and creams on the hair. Once the hair is finally cleansed, natural oils are also washed away from the hair leaving it dryer than it was before.

Use products for your hair texture and or scalp issue: Products that work on one person doesn't necessarily work on another. If you want fullness, use a volumizing shampoo and conditioner along with maintenance products that make the hair appear fuller. If you want to remove product build up, use cleansers such as clarifying or purifying shampoo to remove oil and dirt. These products will contain surfactants (ingredient that attract oil and dirt so it can be washed away) such as ammonium laurel sulfates which is a detergent. To add moisture to the hair, use moisturizing shampoos that contain may panthenol, hydrolized silk, keratin protein or sulfate free ingredients such as sodium lauroyl methyl isethionate. These are examples of ingredients that aid in moisturizing the hair.

Get a trim every 6 -8 weeks: Holding on to things that are not working for you is unhealthy whether it's in life or has something to do with the hair. When the ends of the hair are damaged, the hair breaks resulting in the appearance of slow growth and will cause the splitting to move up the hair shaft creating shedding. If the hair is trimmed on a regular basis, less hair will shed and more length will be achieved. Contrary to what some people think, the hair grows from the root and not the ends. Besides, holding on to split ends for length went out in the 80's and remember, the longer you wait, the more hair that has to be cut unless you find a stylist that will show mercy on the first visit.

Get protein treatments every 8 weeks: This treatment strengthens the bonds in the hair that may be damaged from chemicals such as color and relaxers, heat styling, extensions or rough handling while the hair is wet. It is not necessary to treat the hair more than two months because excessive use will harden the hair resulting in possible breakage.

Oil the scalp about once a week for natural styles: after a few days it's not uncommon for a little dryness to settle in so oiling the scalp would bring relief from itching. For fine textures, use lighter oils such as sesame, grape seed, or coconut. For medium and coarse textures use heavier oils such as jojoba, avocado, or almond. Any combination of these oils would also be good to use. Each individual have to use what works for them. If you are wearing your hair straight, it's not necessary to oil the scalp because this will weigh the hair down causing it to lose its bounce and become stiff.

Take the time to care for the hair that grows out of your head: The truth usually hurts, but here it is. Weaves and extensions are fine, but don't get to the point where the only reason to wear extensions is to hide damaged hair and missing edges. Shoes, hand bags, and someone else's DNA in the form of hair in a bag all seem to be more of a priority over proper hair care so go to the salon, get trims and treatments or some kind of hair care regimen that will keep the hair healthy. Being natural doesn't always mean you have to do it yourself.

Don'ts:

Don't wear extensions past 8-12 weeks: 12 weeks is really pushing it because there will be a lot of new growth after that amount of time. Wearing weaves too long will cause the hair to mildew and or dry rot from being wet in a braided state for long periods after shampooing. It is imperative for the overall health of the hair so shampoo it every two weeks while wearing extensions to avoid a situation such as this. Also, sit under the dryer long enough to dry the extensions.

Don't braid or put a weave on relaxed hair: The bonds in the hair have already been broken down with the chemical and the hair is at its weakest point. Therefore putting additional tension on the hair can cause further damage which won't be seen until the braids are taken out.

Don't put water on hair that has been braided or twisted without brushing it out: Doing so will result in excessive tangling and matting causing more breakage as the hair is combed out.

Don't comb the hair roughly when it is wet: The hair is weakest while wet so it should be combed gently to avoid breakage. If the hair is damaged during the combing process, it will tangle when wet especially if it's long.

Don't put oil on the hair: Oil on the hair can actually dry it out because it sits on the hair shaft and doesn't penetrate to moisturize. Plus, when the hair is shampooed, the oil that was applied and the hair's natural oils are stripped away making the hair dry.

Don't wait until the hair looks bad before getting it done: Not only is it country, it's downright ridiculous! Why would you hold on to the same hair style for weeks just because it doesn't look bad? You're creating more work for the stylist when you wait and the hair is suffering from neglect. By the time you get to the salon, there's dandruff, dry scalp, tangling, dry hair, you name it. A regular routine would eliminate some of these issues. And for the record, we as stylists don't want your flakes all over our floor, clothes and equipment. Yeah I said it!

Glossary

Ammonium laurel Sulfate - is a high foam surfactant that allows water to easily penetrate the hair for deeper cleaning. Simply put, it is a cleanser

Ammonium laureth Sulfate - a foaming agent that works as a detergent and surfactant

Ammonium Thioglycolate - free ammonia that swells the hair rendering it permeable once applied. This is the chemical found in perm solution

Antioxidants - substances that protect cells from damage caused by unstable molecules called free radicals

Apoptosis - the process of cell death and happens during the catagen phase of the hair growth cycle

Atom - Smallest amount of an element that make up for everyday objects

Calcium Hydroxide - a mixture of calcium oxide (lime) and water which is also caustic (poisonous) and is used in cement, industrial solvents and cleaners, no lye hair straighteners

Ceteareth-30 - A surfactant used as an emulsifier which is an emulgent (allows two unblendable substances to become stable in their blended state)

Cetyl Alcohol - Derived from plants; it works as an emulsifier, emollient, thickener and carrying agent in cosmetic solutions. Also a fatty alcohol derived from coconut oil and palm oil. As an emulsifier it helps oil and water mix

Citric Acid - Classified as a weak organic acid, it is a natural preservative and acts as a pH (power of hydrogen) adjuster in hair and skin care products. The hair's normal pH is 5.5; anything less than 7 is acid and anything higher than 7 is alkaline

Compound - Molecule containing more than one element

Element - Basic substance that cannot be simplified

Formaldehyde - Colorless strong-smelling gas often found in water based solutions. It is used as a preservative in medical laboratories and mortuaries and used in products such as glue, household products, and chemicals

Free Radicals - reactive chemicals that can harm cells at high concentrations

Hydrolysis - Reaction with water involving the breaking of a bond in a molecule

Keratin - a protein found in the skin, nails and hair

Methylene Glycol - The reaction of formaldehyde with water produces methylene glycol which can be found in hair straighteners like Brazilian Blow Out

Mineral Oil - is liquid petroleum created through a distillation process which is a method used to separate substances. The process involves converting liquid into vapor and condensing it back to liquid. Petroleum produce gasoline which comes from crude oil (from crude oil you get gasoline, from gasoline you get petroleum, from petroleum you get mineral oil. What determines the quality of the mineral oil is how refined it is so it won't clog pores

Molecule - Two or more atoms chemically joined together

Organic - Matter that has come from a once living organism

Panthenol - Form of vitamin B5 (alcohol analog of pantothenic acid) and used as a lubricating compound and moisturizer.

Pantothenic Acid - Water soluble vitamin known as B5 found in plants and animals.

Paraben - A preservative used to prevent the growth of bacteria in cosmetic products.

Petrolatum - a byproduct of petroleum which is a combination of oil and natural gas

pH - Stands for potential hydrogen and is measured by its hydrogen ion concentration of any solution. The lower the pH, the more acidic and oxygen deprived the fluid is and the higher the pH, the more alkaline and oxygen rich the fluid is. The pH scale is measured from 1-14; anything below 7.0 is acidic and anything above 7.0 is alkaline with 7.0 being neutral. For those that still relax the hair, remember that the pH balance of the hair is 5.5 therefore a normalizing shampoo should be used to restore the hair to is proper pH, a neutralizing shampoo will only bring the hair to 7.0 after relaxing. The body cannot heal itself in an acidic state and if the body's pH isn't balanced, food supplements, vitamins and minerals are not effective.

Protein - is made up of amino acids which are organic compounds that the body uses to make proteins that help with functions that include hair growth. A strand of hair is made up of protein therefore requiring protein in order to grow

Silk - A natural protein fiber

Sodium Benzoate - a preservative that has the "ability to deprive cells of oxygen, break down the immune system and cause cancer" (naturalnew.com 2014)
for cells to function properly and fight off infection, they require oxygen which sodium benzoate deprives them of that

Sodium Hydroxide - poisonous chemical known as lye or caustic soda. It's found in drain cleaners, metal polishers, oven cleaners, and hair straighteners also known as relaxer

Sodium lauroyl methyl isethionate - a sulfate free surfactant derived from coconut oil used as a mild cleanser

Surfactant - a combination of organic compounds lipophilic (oil attracting) and hydrophilic (water attracting) agents that washes away oil and dirt

References

Hair Science. (2016, June 16) Retrieved from http://www.hair-science.com/_int/_en/index.aspx

WebMD. (2014, July 2) Retrieved from http://www.webmd.com/skin-problems-and-treatments/hair-loss/

American Hair Loss Association. (2014, July 2) Retrieved from http://www.americanhairloss.org/types_of_hair_loss/

JW Salon Styles. (2013, November 25) Retrieved from http://www.jwsalonstyles.com/

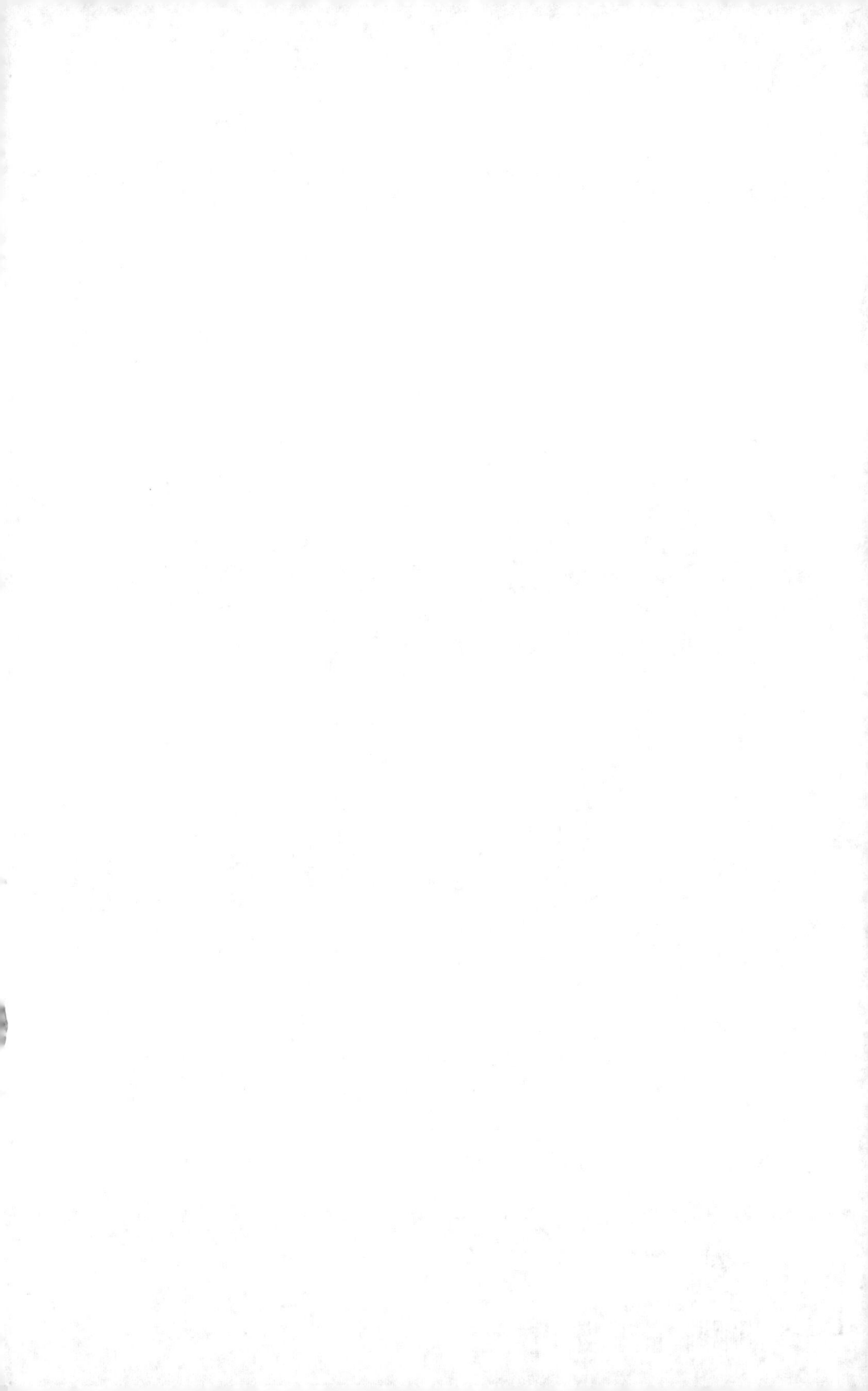

www.ingramcontent.com/pod-product-compliance
Lightning Source LLC
Chambersburg PA
CBHW062118280526
45788CB00003B/1506